Giant-Cell Arteritis

One Man's Exciting Experience

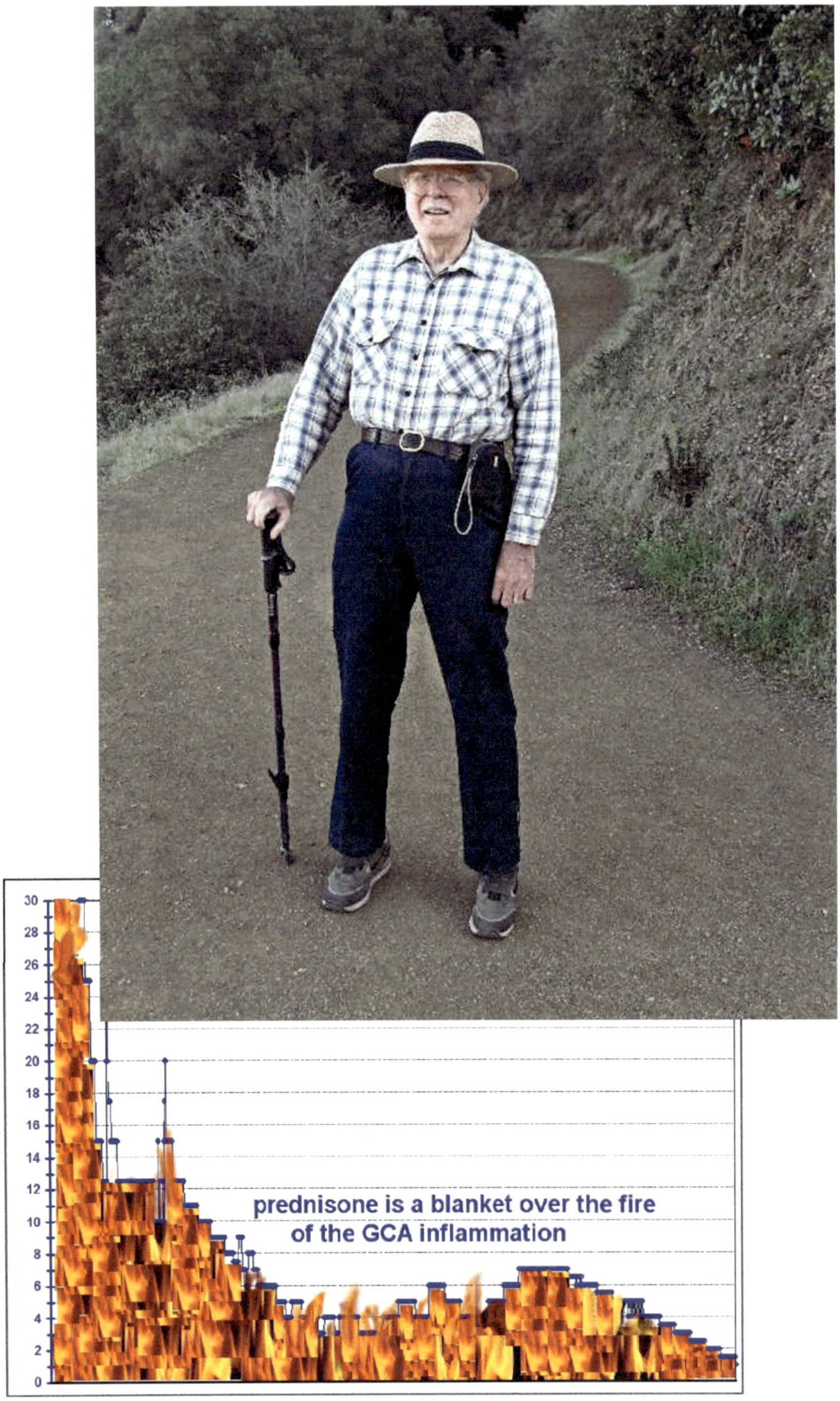
30
28
26
24
22
20
18
16
14
12
10
8
6
4
2
0
prednisone is a blanket over the fire
of the GCA inflammation

Giant-Cell Arteritis

One Man's Exciting Experience

updated August 2016

Mason A. Clark

The Frontal Lobe ®
Los Altos, California

GCA-222rev.wpd

This is an August 2016 update of the 2012 edition.
Graphs are updated and improved; the text refined.

There may be continuing updates, additions, or changes displayed at my website::

http://frontal-lobe.info/gca/gca.html

Comments, criticisms, and reviews will be welcomed.
Modern printing makes editing quite feasible.

ISBN : 978-0931400-05-6

Printed in the United States of America

Published by Frontal Lobe®
http://frontal-lobe.info
Los Altos, California

Preface

Important -- Read this first !

This is the story of one man's Giant-Cell Arteritis. GCA is not life-shortening, not painful, and is readily treatable, but starts as an emergency requiring immediate treatment. If you are suspected of having GCA you will be treated immediately, awaiting diagnosis details. This book describes what for me has been a fascinating GCA experience. It should be both encouraging and instructive.

I am not a medical doctor. Some of my understandings of my own experience may differ from that of my doctor – and may differ from that of your doctor. There are some controversies that medical practice will work out in due time..

This is simply one patient's experience with GCA including reading of the medical literature and of the experiences of other GCA and PMR patients.

If you have GCA, enjoy the excitement – you might as well because it is not going to be quickly cured. It will go into remission in its own time. For me, GCA has been a fun hobby from age 88 to 95 and continuing.

Comments, criticism, reviews, errors and thanks will be appreciated.
masonc@frontal-lobe.info Web site: Frontal-Lobe.info

Table of Contents

Illustrations

Giant-Cell Arteritis
also known as Temporal Arteritis

What is GCA ("Temporal Arteritis") ?

"Giant cell arteritis (GCA) is an inflammation of the lining of your arteries -- the blood vessels that carry oxygen-rich blood from your heart to the rest of your body. Most often, it affects the arteries in your head, especially those in your temples. For this reason, giant cell arteritis is sometimes called temporal arteritis or cranial arteritis. "Giant cell arteritis frequently causes headaches, jaw pain, and blurred or double vision. Blindness and, less often, stroke are the most serious complications of giant cell arteritis. "Prompt treatment with corticosteroid medications usually relieves symptoms of giant cell arteritis and may prevent loss of vision. You should start feeling better within days of starting your treatment."

Mayo Clinic staff

Caution: GCA is a systemic inflammation of certain kinds of arteries anywhere, not only on the head.

Diagnosis of GCA

The American College of Rheumatology recommends that GCA be diagnosed if *three* of the following *five* are true:

Age is 50 or older
New, localized headache
Temporal artery tenderness or decreased pulse
Blood test: erythrocyte sedimentation rate, ESR, greater than 50 mm/hr
Temporal-artery biopsy positive for GCA

An additional, strong clue is the very quick relief of symptoms by taking prednisone, usually in one or two days.

It is universally agreed that if GCA is suspect, prednisone should be given immediately to prevent some loss of vision in one eye. A strong dose of prednisone for a few days is relatively harmless and a relief of symptoms in one or two days is an almost certain diagnosis of GCA.

GCA Symptoms

1. Weight loss
2. Fatigue
3. Malaise: The feeling of overall ill health and weakness.
4. Constitutional symptoms: In this subset of GCA, the disease process. is dominated by manifestations of system-wide inflammation, including rise in ESR and/or CRP
5. Headaches: throbbing, sharp or dull headaches may bring you to your doctor.
6. Tenderness near the temples: Noticed most when wearing glasses, combing hair or lying on a pillow.
7. Fever: Spiking temperature and chills will bring you to the doctor. Or low-grade fever
8. Loss of appetite
9. Jaw claudication: pain, tension and weakness of the muscles that allow you to chew and talk.
10. Less common: Tongue, throat and neck pain
11. Amaurosis fugax: A fleeting visual blurring with heat or exercise, or posture-related visual blurring; it may precede partial or complete blindness and requires an emergency visit to the doctor.
12. Double vision (diplopia)
13. Blindness: Loss of vision is sudden, painless and usually permanent.
14. Dry cough (a cough is not often listed as a symptom of GCA but has been reported)

Polymyalgia Rheumatica (PMR)

PMR is a cousin affliction of GCA. Its name in English is "many muscle pains" and it is treated with prednisone in much the same way as GCA. About 50% of patients with GCA also have PMR. About 20% of patients with PMR also have GCA. The reason is unknown. PMR is painful but is not regarded as dangerous. GCA is a threat to vision and to large arteries such as the aorta. Both are treated successfully with prednisone. Neither are cured but usually subside by themselves in time..

I have GCA but have not experienced PMR so I will not write about PMR.

The similarity of treatment and the possibility of a PMR patient developing GCA makes this booklet instructive for PMR patients.

GCA patients must be aware of the possibility of having or getting PMR.

PMR Symptoms

These are listed by the Mayo Clinic:

Aches or pain in your shoulders (often the first symptom)
Aches or pain in your neck, lower back, buttocks, hips or thighs
Tenderness in your upper arms
Stiffness in affected areas, particularly in the morning
Limited range of motion in affected areas
Pain or stiffness in wrists or knees (less common)
Low-grade fever. Fatigue – A general feeling of not being well (malaise)
Loss of appetite. Unintended weight loss. Depression

My GCA Diagnosis

Warnings: I had several unusual health experiences in the six months before my GCA crisis. Were they related to GCA? Did one or the other induce GCA? I don't know. The cause of GCA is unknown.

An ear infection, only time in my life. Antibiotics cured it.
A red eye, only time in my life. It subsided in a week or two.
A loss of weight from about 183 to about 173. Unusual for me
A rising resting heart rate from 72 to 90 over a three-month period.
A brief incident of double vision, the date was not recorded.

I was not otherwise aware of a health problem during this time until a dry cough sent me to a pulmonary doctor. A dry cough is thought to be one of the symptoms of GCA.

The x-ray and CT scan of my lungs did not explain the cough and the diagnosis was "post-nasal drip" but an antibiotic was prescribed "just in case."' The CT scan was done on February 5.

Then, on February 9, 2009 there began a severe headache which on the next day was intense and entirely on the right side. Simultaneously -- on the same day -- there began a severe, persistent constipation – unusual for me.

On February 27 I visited my primary-care physician and had blood tests including ESR (erythrocyte sedimentation rate).

The diagnosis of GCA was made on March 11, 2009 based on severe headaches on the right side and blood tests showing a high ESR of 49. Prednisone was prescribed immediately.. A biopsy of a temporal artery – a simple procedure – was done on March 17, 2009 and confirmed GCA.

A brain MRI and a colonoscopy had been ordered. Neither showed anything important (but the constipation was brought to an abrupt end). I will omit photographs because these tests were not pertinent.

Because of my ignorance and my misunderstanding of the clear instructions of the prescription, I took only 20 mg of prednisone for three days. The headache stopped the day after the first pill. My rheumatologist firmly corrected me and got me started on the correct dosage of 60 mg daily.

> What is "mg"? A milligram. A one-carat diamond weighs 200 milligrams. A common small mosquito weight about 2 ½ mg.
> A one mg prednisone pill is mostly harmless filler to give it manageable size.

Having Fun With GCA and Prednisone

By coincidence or by prednisone euphoria, at this time I discovered the trails of nearby Rancho San Antonio Park. There are miles of trails, mostly in forest, and climbing 200 or 400 or 1000 feet.

I began marking off the trails as I explored them, walking from two to seven miles each day and climbing from 200 to 400 to 1000 feet. Not mountain climbing but great exercise for an 87-year old. Mountain lions are sometimes seen here. Deer and wild turkeys are numerous – as are hikers, joggers, and people. Even old guys with GCA.

Contour Map of Rancho San Antonio Park

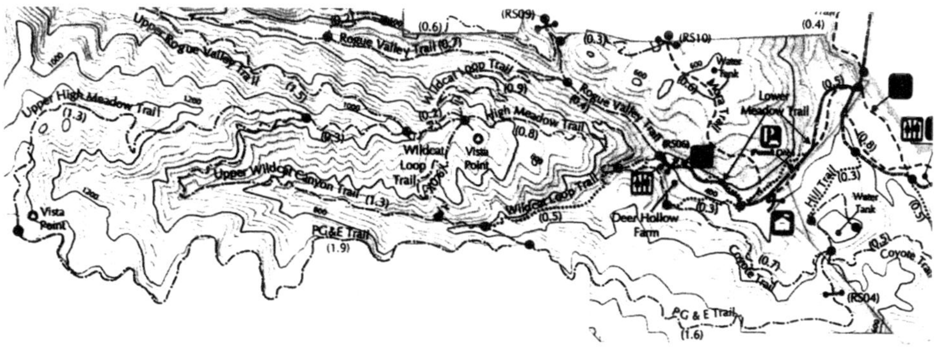

Treatment of GCA -- Prednisone

Note: prednisone is commonly prescribed in the U.S., prednisolone in the U.K. Other variations of prednisone may be prescribed, such as methyl prednisone and hydrocortisone. Coated tablets are sometimes used to minimize stomach irritation. The differences are not important, although the quantities prescribed and schedule of use may differ. For this article, only the word "prednisone" will be used.

Prednisone or other corticosteroids are the only treatment of GCA. Prednisone does not cure the arteritis. It does provide relief from the symptoms and reduces the inflammation. The inflammation is harmful to large, flexible arteries including the large aorta leading from the heart and large leg arteries. It is important that the inflammation be reduced.

The arteritis subsides on its own over a period of time of its own choosing. That time may range from less than a year to two years, five years, or the remainder of lifetime. As time goes on, less prednisone is needed culminating in as little as zero or one milligram per day to as much as 16 mg per day. The small amounts that are common have negligible side effects. The prednisone is not expensive.

GCA is hiding under the carpet of prednisone. The trick is to keep it there with as little prednisone as possible. Good luck.

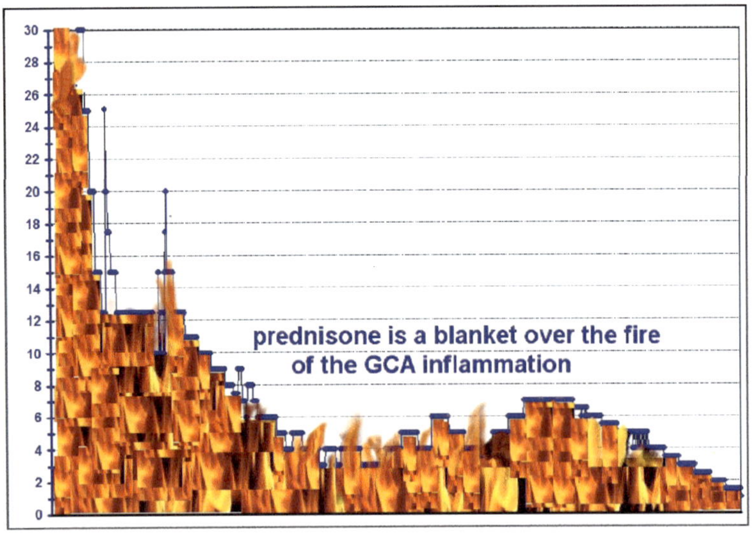

The treatment task is to reduce the prednisone as quickly as possible without permitting a dangerous flare-up of the arteritis. Dangerous because some degree of loss of vision may occur. Too-rapid a withdrawal may also cause a cortisol insufficiency – explained later.

There are three objectives of the treatment:

1. prevent damage to arteries by the GCA inflammation, especially the artery supplying the optic nerve behind the eye. Damage to this nerve causes loss of vision, perhaps complete and irreversible. Leg arteries and the large aorta arteries may also be damaged.
2. minimize prednisone side-effects
3. avoid a crisis of too little cortisol, simulating Addison's disease and dangerous.

GCA may be self-curing but may last from six months to two years or longer. During its life it may do great damage. Treatment is essential. Prednisone wards off the damaging inflamation, giving GCA time to subside, but does not cure GCA. Withdrawal of prednisone is experimental.

Paraphrasing the words of William Blake:

"The road of excess leads to the palace of wisdom. We never know how much is enough until we know how much is not enough."

GCA is hiding under the carpet of prednisone. Lifting the carpet -- withdrawing the prednisone too aggressively -- can let the GCA tiger out. The experience of GCA patients is expressed in the words of Blake:

"Tiger, tiger, burning bright
In the forests of the night,
What immortal hand or eye
Could frame thy fearful symmetry?"

GCA symptoms at this stage may be very subtle or the first warning symptom may by some degree of vision loss. For that reason, caution is required.

In addition to the clue given by symptoms, blood tests are used.

The "sedimentation rate" (ESR) and the C-reactive protein (CRP) measure the GCA activity, but these are affected by other inflamatory events, such as a common cold.

The Management of GCA

Blood Tests -- ESR or PV and CRP

ESR and CRP are measures of inflammation. They support one another. "ESR" is Erythrocyte Sedimentation Rate, measured in mm/hour. "CRP" is C-Reactive Protein, measured in mg/L, sometimes in mg/dL (deciliter). Plasma Viscosity "PV" is occasionally used in place of ESR.

These are the first paragraphs of explanations given on the web site:
http://www.patient.co.uk/doctor/ (on one line)
Acute-Phase-Proteins-CRP-ESR-and-Viscosity.htm

Erythrocyte Sedimentation Rate

"The erythrocyte sedimentation rate (ESR) measures how fast red cells fall through a column of blood. It is an indirect index of acute phase protein concentrations and is a sensitive but nonspecific index of plasma protein changes which result from inflammation or tissue damage. . . ."

Plasma Viscosity

"Is also a sensitive but nonspecific index of plasma protein changes which result from inflammation or tissue damage. It provides similar information to the erythrocyte sedimentation rate (ESR).

"Increases in parallel with the ESR, but plasma viscosity is not affected by haematocrit variations (e.g. anaemia or polycythaemia) and delay in analysis. It is therefore considered to be vastly under utilized and more reliable than the ESR. . . ."

C-Reactive Protein

"Is an acute phase protein which increases in connective tissue disorders and neoplastic disease. It is increased by bacterial infections and generally less elevated in viral infections.

"C-reactive protein (CRP) is better than erythrocyte sedimentation rate (ESR) for monitoring fast changes as it does not depend on fibrinogen or immunoglobulin levels, and is not affected by red blood cell numbers and shape. These blood tests, along with symptoms, guide treatment. . . ."

"Normal" Healthy Values of ESR

What are normal values for ESR? The Norwegians have collected data from 3910 healthy Norwegian adults, most of whom were healthy blood donors. Their data displayed in the chart below shows that more than 84% of men and 66% of women of all ages have a normal ESR less than eight (8).

Healthy ESR Values

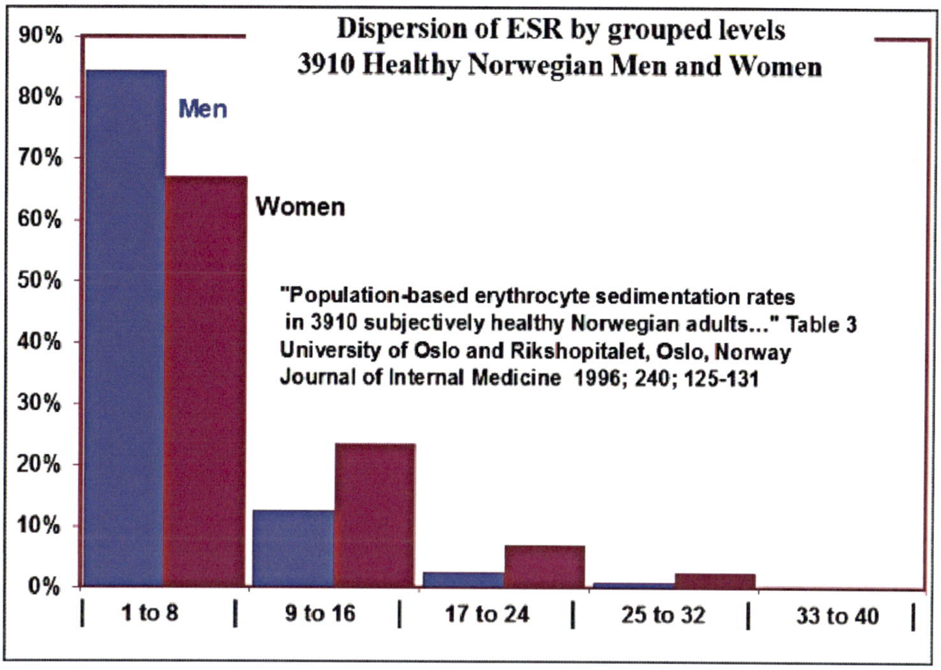

If 20 is used as a limit considered normal, then a person with a healthy ESR of 4 who has an ESR of 17 would be called "normal." This could lead to error in treatment. With or without symptoms it would warn of inflammation damage being done. The same is true of CRP.

The medical literature has many examples of surprise expressed that a patient with such a "normal" ESR blood test has GCA.

A common statement is, "Patients with GCA frequently experience unpredictable relapses; however, an isolated increase of ESR or CRP in the absence of symptom is not cause for increasing the prednisone dosage."

The first symptom of an "unpredictable relapse" may be loss of vision from one eye. The experience of an ophthalmology department will be given later.

Increase of ESR with Age

ESR increases with age, but not by a misleading formula often quoted. The graph below shows the Norwegian data and the old formula.

For ages 55 to 90 – that of patients with GCA:

> For men the average ESR is 5 to 10.
> 95% of healthy men are below 14 to 18.
>
> For women the average ESR is 8 to 11.
> 95% of healthy women are below 21 to 23.

So it is reasonable for a laboratory to post a red flag to get the doctor's attention when the ESR is over 20. However, an individual might have an ESR of 4 when healthy and an ESR of 12 would be high.

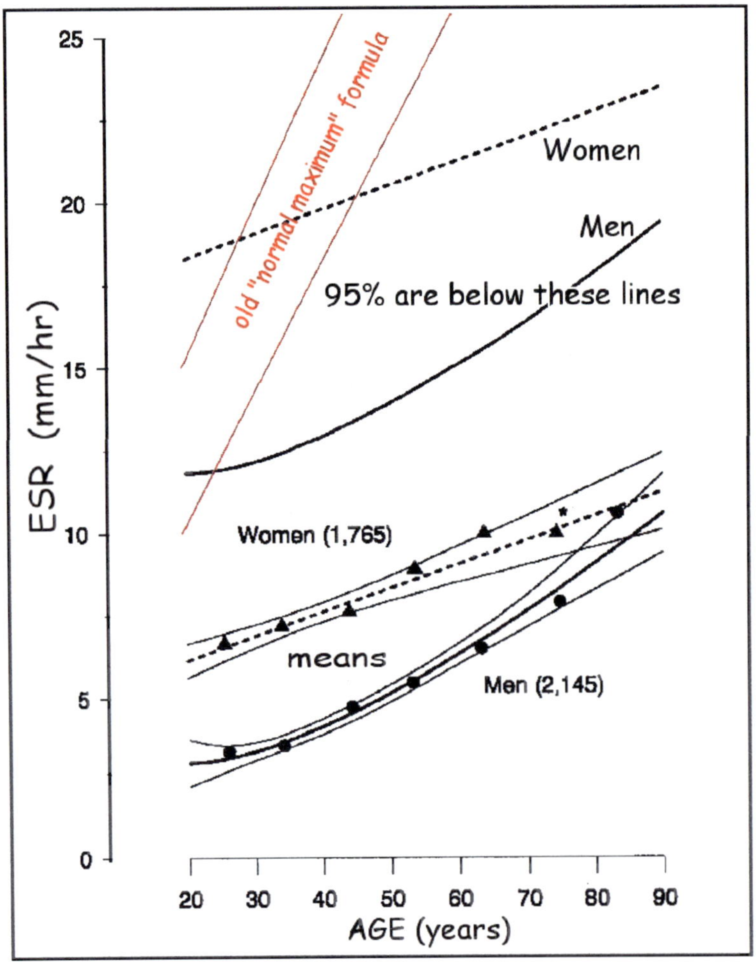

The ESR and CRP can Mislead

ESR and CRP are not specific for GCA and PMR. They are elevated by other inflammations. The common cold, influenza, and urinary track infections raise their values.

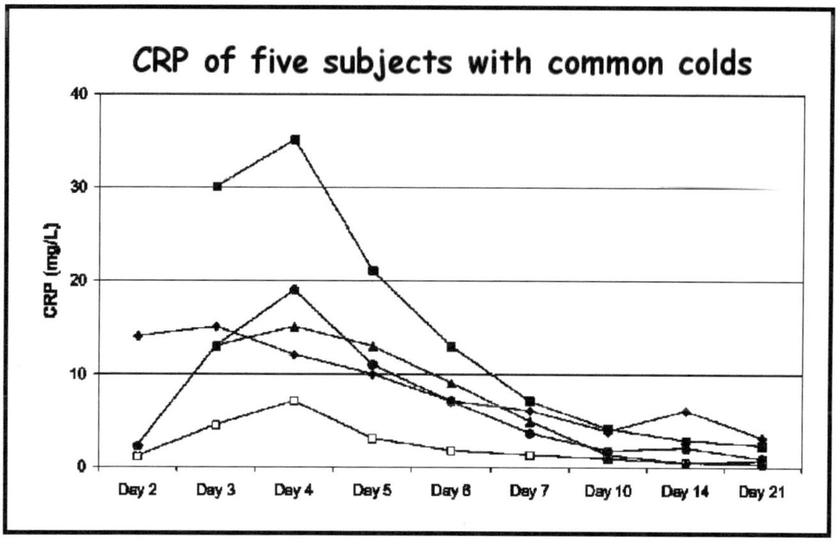

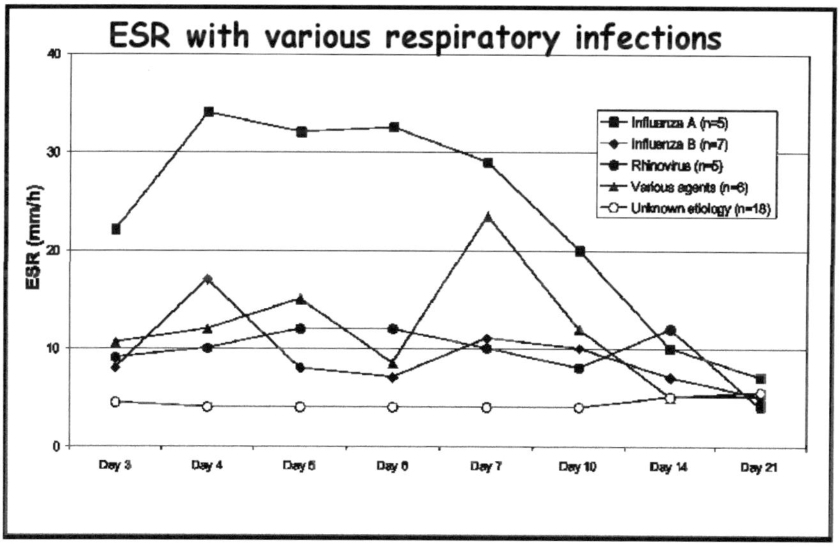

When Normal is not Normal

It is essential to recognize that a person with a normal ESR of four (4) who is found to have an ESR of 14 may have serious GCA inflammation. And this is in spite of the fact that the ESR of 14 is below the laboratory's and doctor's warning only when ESR is over 20.

Prolonged, unsuppressed inflammation is damaging to the arteries and represents a condition when an unpleasant and even dangerous flare may happen.

Unlike most blood test numbers, ESR and CRP vary over a wide range. These are reactions to inflammation and may range from almost zero to a high number, perhaps more than 100.

What is "normal" for the population is not the correct guide for judging the numbers for an individual.

As the Norwegian article says:

"There is obviously an important difference between subject-based and population-based ESR values.

"There are two ways of establishing the upper reference limit for an individual ESR test. The ESR can be statistically calculated from a population based ESR taking into consideration the extra uncertainty associated with a single test, as presented in this study.

"Another, and more valid method is to determine personal baseline values for each individual. Kjeldsberg says that ESR readings `may be especially helpful when the test results are compared with baseline values for the individual patient .'

"At the moment we have no collection of statistical data on subject-based time series in healthy persons, but one of the authors has recorded his ESR at frequent intervals from the age of 30 to 72. Apart from short periods of fever and, and a serious attack of cholecystitis (ESR 90 mm/hr), his ESR has fluctuated between 1 and 4 mm/hr, with 2 mm/hr as an average. For such a person a level of 15 mm/hr would mean an increase of more than 800%, but it would still be below the population-based upper reference limit for the age of 70.

"Griffiths *et al* have also found that many ESR values fall below the upper reference limit in many people, even with disease. Hence, the individually most valid reference is each patient's baseline value judged on the basis of serial recordings. A single ESR measurement which is either above the upper population-based reference limit or, even better, above the personal mean baseline should cause clinical concern and lead to control tests, and for further investigations."

A common error that appears in the medical literature is represented by a statement such as:

"Ten of 177 (6%) patients had normal ESR values at diagnosis (< or = 30 mm/hr)."

Here "normal ESR" was defined as 30 or less. But what was the healthy normal of each of those ten patients? Perhaps it was 3 and they had 23 and were definitely suffering from inflammation.

A patient tells us: "My ESR and CRP tests were normal so my prednisone dose was reduced from 9 mg to 8 mg and a relapse occurred." The "normal" was the population normal, not the normal of this patient. One only hopes the resultant relapse was not serious.

Articles from the University of Iowa Hospital ophthalmology department instruct:

"..the only trustworthy and safe parameters to regulate the steroid therapy and to prevent visual loss are the levels of ESR and CRP, and nothing else."

The blood tests, ESR and CRP – along with symptoms – give us instruction for the management of the prednisone. The new patient and doctor will not know the patient's normal ESR and CRP. The normals for the population do not apply. They are an aid in diagnosis but useless in managing the prednisone for a particular patient. The individual's normal can only be learned by observation as treatment proceeds.

Dr. Hunder, Professor Emeritus at the Mayo Clinic College of Medicine recommends:

"Results of ESR and CRP testing should be interpreted in the context of the patient's typical values prior to the onset of illness, when available, and the patient's age."

The patient's healthy ESR and CRP are rarely available and must be learned from the lowest values seen during treatment. It is essential to understand that the population normal so often mentioned may be dangerously misleading in the on-going treatment of an individual.

Controversy: An Ophthalmology Department Speaks

Rheumatologists have experience with the serious side effects of prednisone and are rightly anxious to reduce the amount of prednisone.

Ophthalmologists are, by profession, anxious to prevent loss of vision, a too-common effect of GCA. The Ophthalmologist, Dr. Hayreh, has concluded from extensive experience:

"In my studies of about 300 patients with GCA, I found that the only way to manage GCA to prevent blindness is to regulate the therapy and management is by doing ESR and GCA regularly. Rheumatologists advocate that the therapy should be regulated by symptoms only, which I have found totally wrong and dangerous strategy. Symptoms are no guide to the activity of GCA. I have a large number of patients in whom ESR and CRP went sky high without recurrence of systemic symptoms. I have seen patients who were managed by rheumatologists with that outlook coming to me with loss of vision. Thus, the only way to prevent blindness due to GCA is by ESR and CRP estimations." (e-mail letter to me)

The graph below shows the experience of 145 patients at the University of Iowa Hospital. My prednisone experience is superimposed.

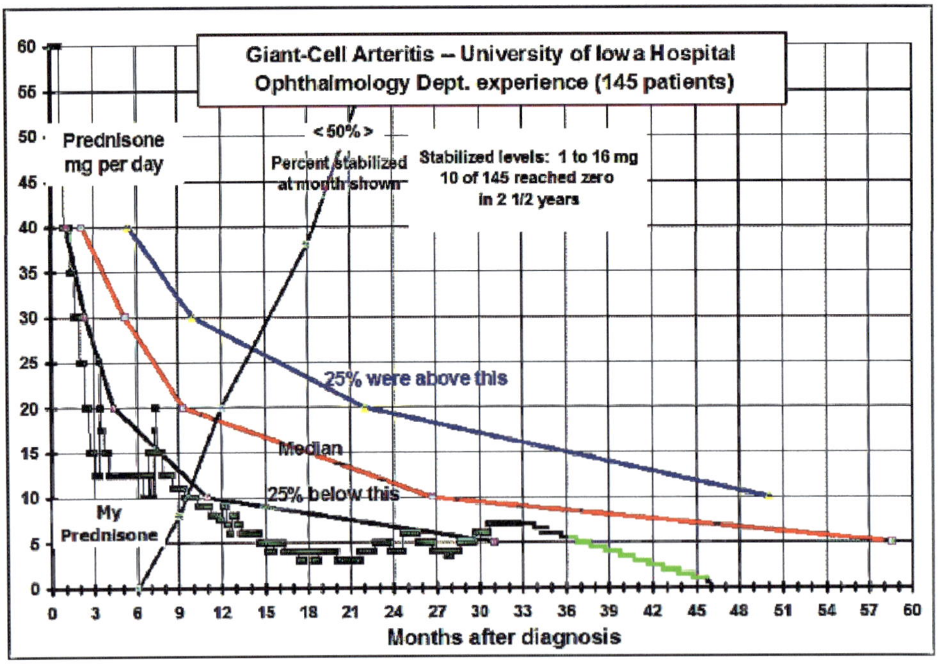

Notice:

1. The amount and length of time for the use of prednisone.
2. Of 145 patients, only 10 discontinued prednisone.
3. The others settled at maintenance levels from one to sixteen mg.
4. At 24 months, 40% had not yet stabilized at a maintenance level

The side effects of prednisone are a matter of concern. Avoiding flares by cautious reduction of prednisone reduces the total amount of prednisone used. Treating GCA is a slow process, perhaps for the rest of one's life. However – for most patients – the small, maintenance dose of prednisone has little or no side-effects. One can live a comfortable, normal life.

Reading Time Graphs

Examine the simple graph below. Along the bottom is a time scale with dates from left to right. On the side is a scale of something interesting, perhaps the amount of prednisone you are taking each day. Looking up from any date, read the value on the left. – in this example, nine milligrams of prednisone on January 21, 2010.

Read the graph by following the line from left to right – see how it travels as time goes by. A graph of prednisone, ESR, and CRP against time is a valuable aid to GCA prednisone management. Blank graph paper is at the back of this book.

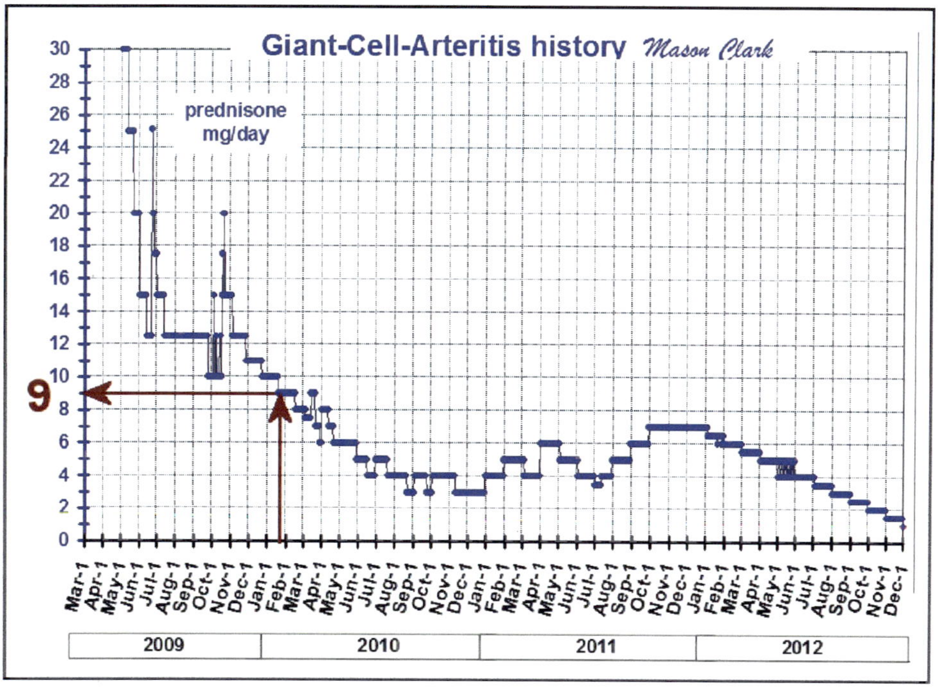

Data is Valuable

Laboratory tests taken over a period of time can be presented as a list of numbers as show here.

This chart is – to me -- a blur of numbers. I cannot see the trends. The course of events is not obvious. I could not use this list as a guide for prednisone treatment.

On the opposite page the top graph is a display of this data. The trends and the dangerous rise to a peak are obvious. There is also a strangely sharp peak near the right of the ESR chart.

Name	ESR
Standard Range	*0.0-20.0 mm/hr*
2/27/2009	50 H
3/9/2009	49 H
4/14/2009	4
6/8/2009	11
8/18/2009	7
10/16/2009	15
11/24/2009	7
12/8/2009	5
1/26/2010	17
3/2/2010	9
3/31/2010	15
4/29/2010	10
5/27/2010	6
6/28/2010	16
7/28/2010	10
8/31/2010	22 H
9/29/2010	17
10/29/2010	13
11/29/2010	16
12/29/2010	18
1/28/2011	14
3/2/2011	15
3/30/2011	36 H
5/2/2011	15
5/31/2011	12
6/30/2011	12
7/27/2011	20
8/27/2011	16
9/26/2011	19
10/27/2011	13
11/28/2011	11
12/26/2011	25 H
12/29/2011	10
2/15/2012	10
3/15/2012	9

Graphs of Data are Better

The clinic I go to believes in graphs. Here are some they provide, printed from their computer's display. The dashed lines are the laboratory's limits for warning of abnormality based on statistics of the healthy population – not my statistics.

ESR, a measure of inflammation. The initial very high value. The rise upward for a time to an abrupt peek, then downwards as GCA subsides.

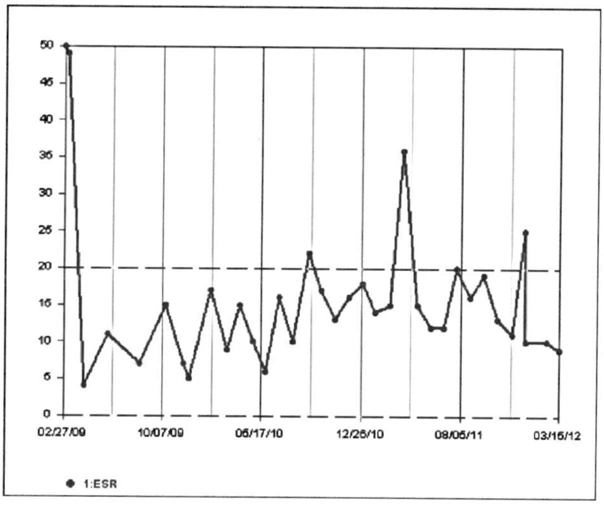

CRP, the other measure of inflammation remained low until a serious rise of inflammation – also shown by ESR. Notice that CRP did not confirm that strangely sharp ESR peak on the right. It was a laboratory error corrected three days later. Without the graphs that error might have misled.

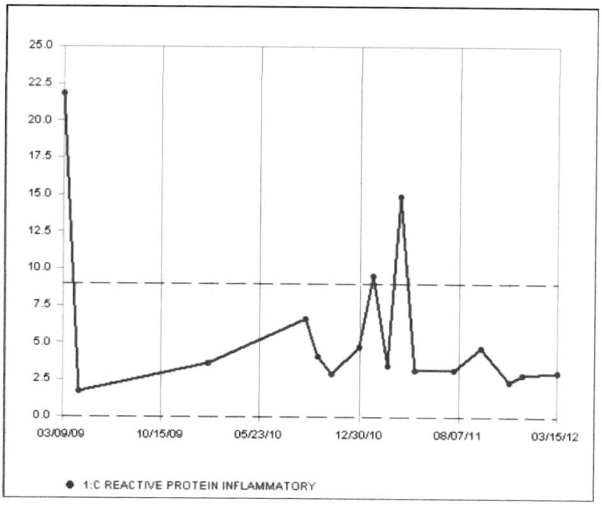

On the following page, these two graphs have been combined.

Finding My "Normal" ESR and CRP

Looking at the lows on the graph below, my normal ESR appears to be between 4 and 10, perhaps 7. The values above ten were certainly not normal for me.

My normal CRP must be less than 2.9. (The lab usually reported "less than 2.9" -- its test limit.) The values of CRP above four were certainly not normal for me. They confirmed the ESR indication of inflammation.

Laboratories tag test numbers to call the doctor's attention to abnormal values. For ESR, 20 is a common level to be tagged. It is not the number to use in treatment of an individual whose normal in good health is almost certainly lower. A patient with a healthy ESR of 2 is certainly not "normal" with an ESR of 12.

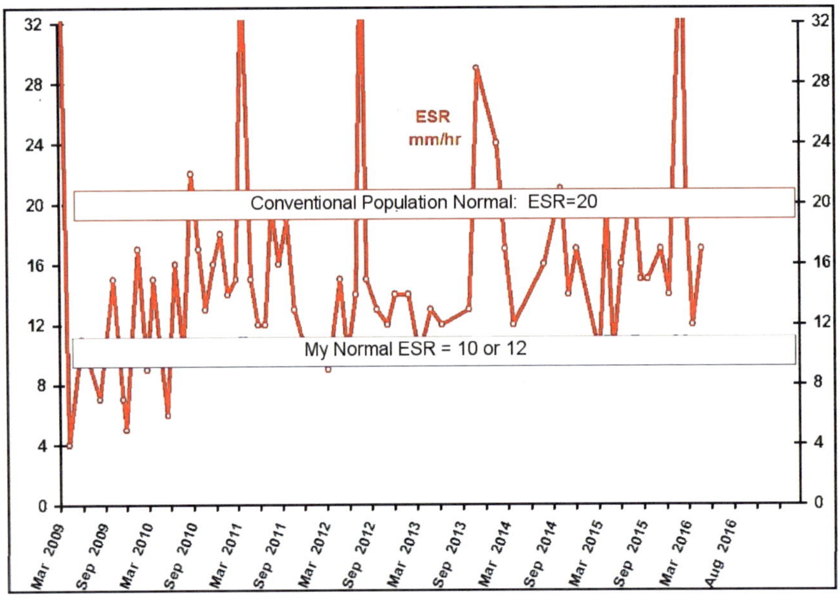

At the early ESR of 15, I had a flare with two temporal arteries swollen that could have cost me some loss of vision if one had been an optic-nerve artery.

During the times of ESR numbers above ten, there were weak, fleeting head-pain symptoms -- symptoms that could be denied, but the numbers revealed the inflammation. I erred by ignoring both these symptoms and my ESR.

Inflammation of my leg arteries brought the day when the ESR and CRP both screamed "STOP" and I stopped prednisone withdrawal, perhaps barely in time to save my legs from more serious artery inflammation. We'll never know, but such inflammation does the arteries no good (see Appendix II).

A Paradox: More Prednisone may be Less Prednisone

Some articles on PMR and GCA assert that "a rise in ESR or CRP does not justify a change of corticosteroid therapy."

But they also say , "a high relapse rate that may be caused by rapid reduction of prednisone leads to an increased cumulative dose and subsequent adverse events."

In addition to possible "adverse events," the flare let loose by a too-fast reduction forces the use of more prednisone after the damage is done.

Avoiding flares by the slow reduction of prednisone may actually result in the use of **less** prednisone. Slow reduction, using the blood tests as a guide minimizes symptoms. A flare is not a warning but is a symptom too late.

GCA Need Not Stop Exercise

Exercise is important – is essential. Here is my photograph taken from the top of Rancho's P G & E trail. The view is of The City of San Jose in the Silicon Valley hiding under clouds. In the distance is Mount Hamilton. It is 1,000 foot climb on an eight -mile walk. The date was August 30, 2009 and I was on 12 ½ mg of prednisone after six months of GCA. This was the third time I had visited this site above the clouds since GCA arrived..

PG&E is Pacific Gas and Electric and the lines bring power to the Silicon Valley from a power plant on the coast over the hills behind us.

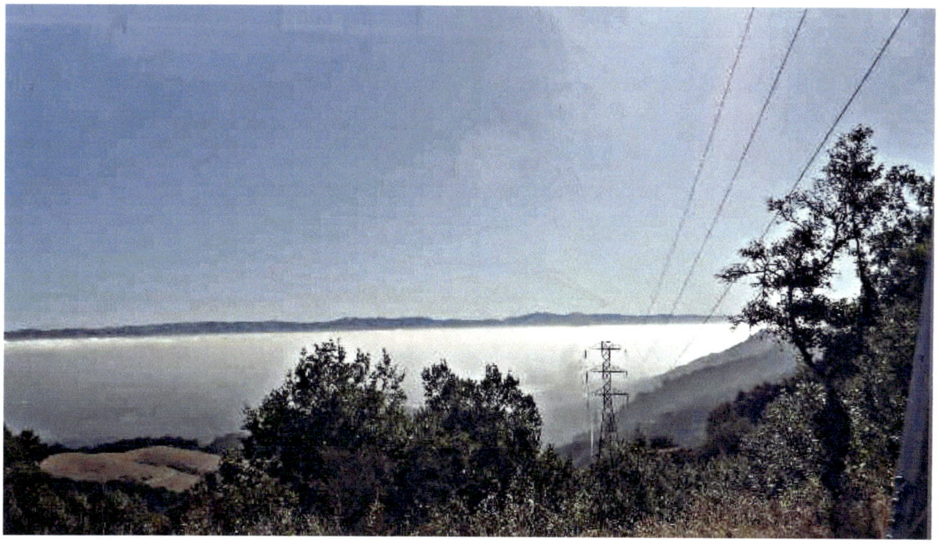

Withdrawal Symptoms: "Addisonian"
Adrenal Cortisol Insufficiency
A crisis

The endocrine system controls the amount of cortisol -- the adrenal cortex hormone -- that is fed to the blood stream. The endocrine system responds to prednisone treatment by reducing the generation of cortisol.

A pathological failure of the adrenal cortex is called "Addison's Disease"

Withdrawal of prednisone too quickly may cause a cortisol deficiency until the adrenal's get back into their business. The symptoms of Addison's disease appear, possibly including a life-threatening crisis.

I experienced from time to time during prednisone withdrawal, these known Addison's warning symptoms:

Sudden penetrating pain in the legs, lower back, or abdomen
Severe lethargy
A general ill feeling
Fever
Loss of appetite
Sensation of vibration in the soles of the feet

Other cortisol insufficiency symptoms include:

Body aches – Abdominal pain – Rapid heart rate – Flank pain, joint pain
Skin rash or lesions
Headaches Nausea or vomiting; dehydration Low blood sugar
Rapid respiratory rate (see tachypnea)
Shaking chills – Slow, sluggish movement
Unusual and excessive sweating on face or palms – Difficulty breathing
Loss of consciousness – Mental changes – Confusion or coma – Salt craving

I had an "Addisonian" crisis on June 22, 2009, after reducing from 15 mg to 12.5 mg.,

Neither I nor my doctor saw this crisis coming although there were warning symptoms for a week.

I had leg pain on Sunday, lethargy all week, no appetite after Thursday. Upon awakening in a sweat the following Monday morning, my sitting or standing blood pressure was 70/50 and I could barely walk.

My doctor ordered me to the emergency ward where I received intra-venous hydro-cortisone and was hospitalized for two nights, June 22 and 23, 2009.

Countless tests confirmed my age of 87 but nothing else to worry about. These tests were necessary for the hospital to rule out other possible causes of my collapse – but at considerable cost (see Appendix III)..

Other than bed rest, intravenous fluid including hydrocortisone – and countless diagnostics – there was no treatment.

The body's normal production of cortisol is said to be 7 mg, so 12.5 mg of prednisone should be sufficient to prevent a shortage crisis.

Prednisone and normal adrenal cortex cortisol hormone production are not one-for-one equivalent, in part because the adrenal cortex provides other hormones, notably aldosterone which is largely responsible for the long-term regulation of blood pressure.

Prednisone Side-Effects

Prednisone side-effects are too numerous to list and discuss here.
I experienced those marked **

** Insomnia (temporarily at highest prednisone levels).

No problem. Just get up and do some work. Or what's on late-night TV? Who needs sleep? I slept 3 hours, worked 3 hours, then slept 2 hours. Then napped 3 hours while watching TV the next day. Missed nothing important.

The insomnia ended when the prednisone was below 20 mg.

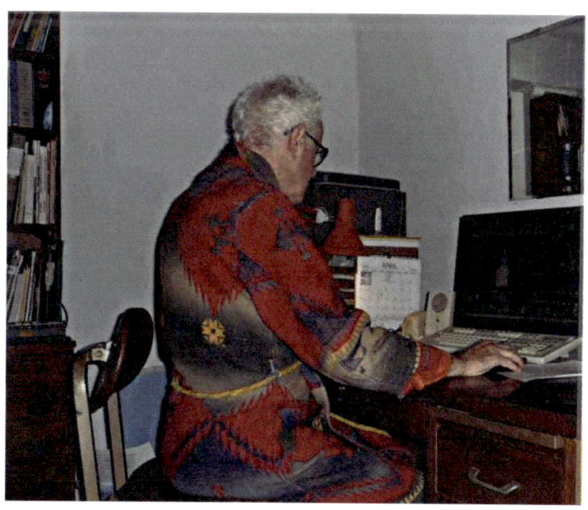

** Fluid retention, causing swelling in lower legs (temporarily at highest prednisone levels) .

** Increased appetite, weight gain -- I recovered only what I had lost .

** Blurred vision, perhaps, like "watering" of eyes.

** Cataracts -- barely perceptible March 2012 after ten grams of prednisone over three years. Cataracts are common in elderly people without prednisone. An ophthalmologist can see these, and they may be removed.

Elevated pressure in the eyes (glaucoma). Tests by an ophthalmologist are imperative. Protective treatment is available.

Increased risk of infections – perhaps the most serious side-effect of suppressing the immune system with prednisone. I had only a common cold which came and went in a normal fashion.

Loss of calcium from bones which can lead to osteoporosis and fractures.
Protective drugs are often prescribed. These have serious side-effects.
An x-ray system called "DEXA" may used to measure bone strength.

Stomach irritation – protective drugs are often prescribed . These have side-effects.

High blood sugar which can trigger or worsen diabetes. Glucose tests are imperative.

Increased blood pressure should be monitored.

Other of the many side-effects include:

Euphoria
Muscle weakness
Mood swings
Thin skin, easy bruising and slower wound healing
Acne
Nervousness, restlessness
Increased growth of body hair
Swollen, "puffy" face
Weight gain; fat deposits abdomen, face, back of neck

Symptoms of GCA, prednisone, and prednisone withdrawal overlap.
It is often difficult to be certain about what is happening.

Home Measurements of Two Prednisone Side-Effects

Blood pressure, resting heart rate, and glucose may be measured with low-priced gadgets from the local drug store. An entertaining feature of mine is the occasional low blood pressure which I sometimes sensed without measurement. It may be a signal of cortisol deficiency.

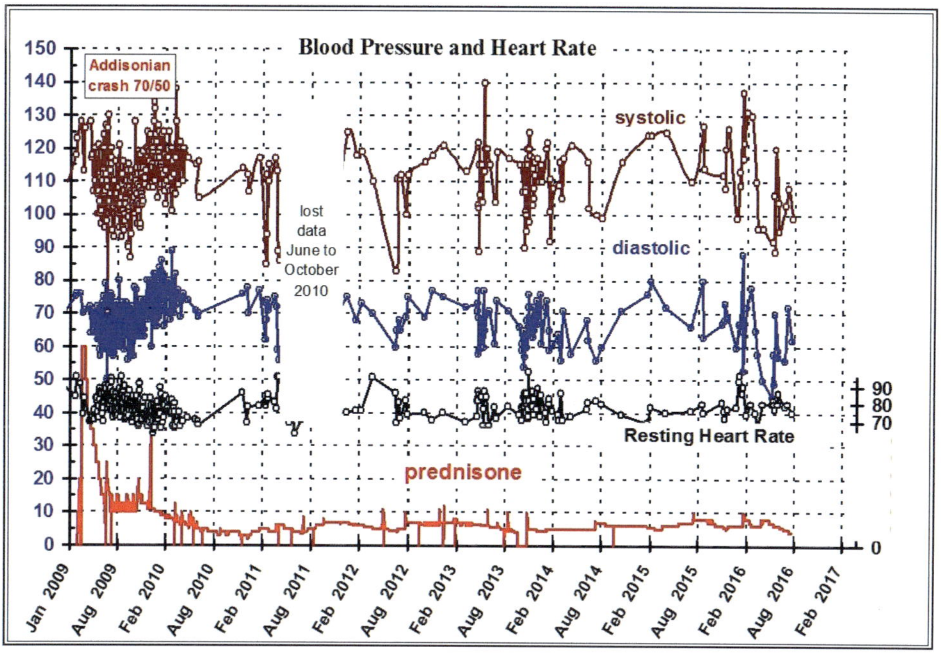

A glucose warning, if there was one, would urge the need for less sugar and white bread and more exercise -- after consultation with your doctor.
My glucose (fasting) had its ups and downs but its trend is favorable.

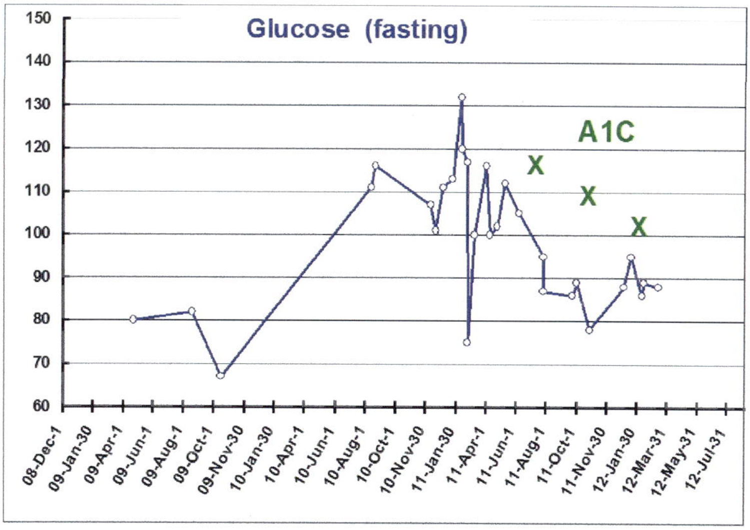

The Instructions of Experience

The following description of my experience is easy to analyze long after the fact. Hindsight is a wonderful tool. Making decisions in real time is far more difficult. Nothing here should be read as a criticism of the decisions of my doctor or myself. We did our best and it has been good enough.

The graph on the opposite page shows my prednisone withdrawal, the rise and fall of ESR and CRP, and three important events.

1. The prednisone level started at 60 mg – off the graph – and was quickly decreased to less than 20 mg.

2. After the drop from 15 mg to 12.5 mg, my sitting/standing blood pressure fell to 70/50 and I required hospitalization and intravenous hydrocortisone.

Intensive testing found nothing else. I left the hospital taking 20 mg but quickly reducing. See Appendix I for more details.

3. From this second 20 mg time a too-rapid decrease to 10 mg led to two right-side temple arteries becoming swollen; one with a spot painful to touch. This flare-up could have struck an artery affecting my vision and demanded a brief return to 12.5 mg.

4. A time at 5, 4, 3, 4, 5 mg continued for more than six months. My symptoms increased, especially leg discomfort (see Appendix II). Therefore I increased to six and then seven mg, and began a careful, slow decrease.

The sed rate, ESR, rose and fell. It may be futile to try to explain each rise and each fall. What is notable is the increase when the prednisone dose fell below 5 mg. The arrows on the graph call attention to this pattern.

Slow Reduction of Prednisone

The often-recommended rule is "no more than 10% at a time." And this usually refers to monthly reductions. At 5 mg only to 4.5 mg which requires cutting the one mg pills. An alternative sometimes used is to alternate between sizes: 5, 4, 5, 4, etc.

Another recommendation is to move gradually to the lower value in this manner: . . 10,10,10,10,10,9,10,10,10,9,10,10,9,10,9,9,10,9,9,9,9,9 . . .

Slowly, gradually is the way to avoid a flare that requires more prednisone.

My GCA History in One Graph

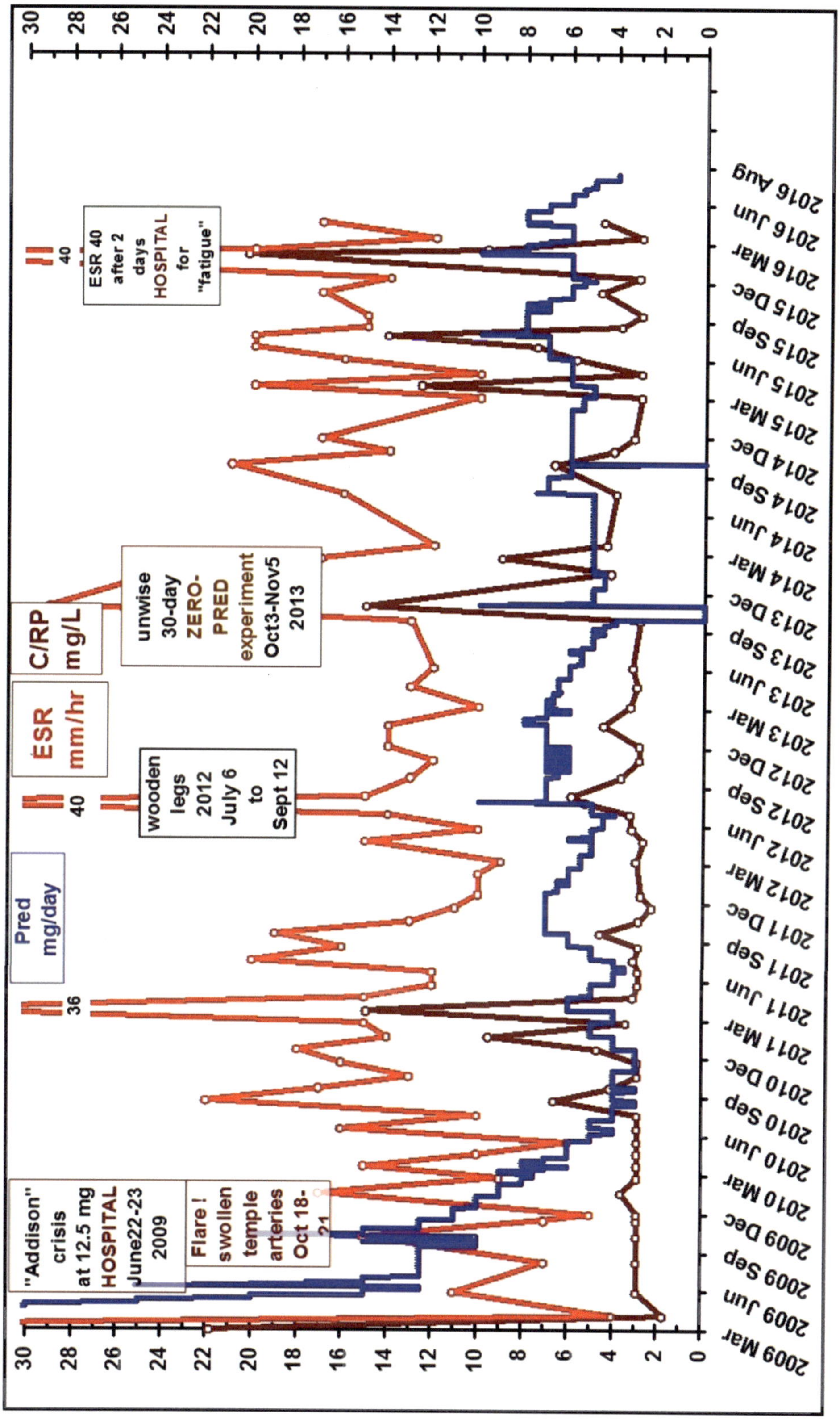

Chronological Summary of My Experience

1. October 5, 2008: I had a "Red-Eye" -- the only one in my life. A Red-Eye is a broken capillary in the white of the eye. It passed in a few days.
2. October to February: my resting heart rose steadily from 72 to 92.

A Warning of Trouble Coming?

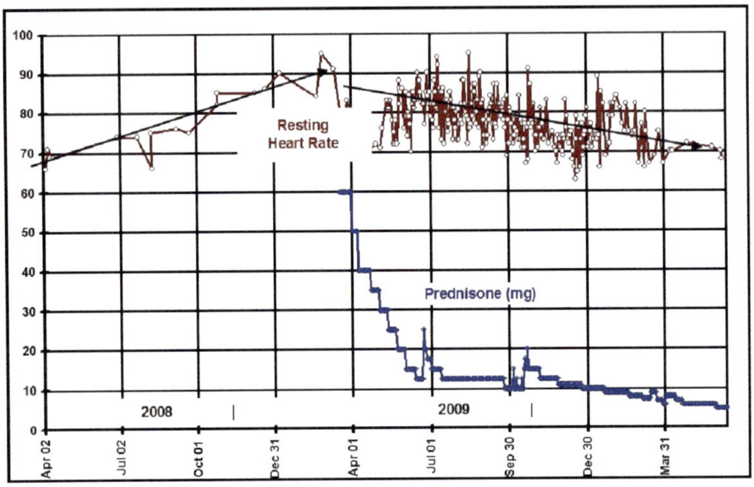

3. My weight fell to 10 pounds below my normal 180.

4. December 22, 2009: I saw a pulmonary doctor about spasms of dry cough and generally not feeling well. I have a history of chronic bronchitis. A chest x-ray showed nothing of immediate importance.

5. February 6, 2009: a CT-scan only showed aging lungs. The diagnosis was "post-nasal drip" but I was given an anti-biotic in case there was an infection.

6. **It really starts** on February 9, 2009: I began a severe night headache on the right side and persistent constipation; both new experiences for me.

7. March 4, 2009: A pulmonary function test showed a normal decline with age.

8. March 9, 2009: I saw my primary-care doctor regarding the headache and constipation.

9. March 11, 2009: A normal MRI brain scan for age 87 -- no brain tumor to account for the one-sided headache.

10. March 11, 2009: the doctor phoned to send me to the pharmacy for prednisone. The lab tests of ESR "sed rate" and CRP had led him immediately to the diagnosis of giant-cell arteritis. This doctor is a geriatrician and GCA is a disease of age over 55. The prescribed prednisone level started at **60 mg** each morning. I misunderstood the prescription and then thought the disappearance of the awful headache meant I had been cured. The rheumatologist forcefully corrected me and got me started on a proper prednisone schedule. I did not take supportive drugs other than calcium and vitamin D.

11. March 12, 2009: the doctor finished my colonoscopy and announced "you don't have cancer" but I had already begun writing my Memoirs.

12. March 17, 2009: a biopsy of a right-temple artery confirmed giant-cell arteritis. My weight had fallen another 8-10 pounds.

13. April 19, 2009: I was feeling well and began the exploration of local hiking trails. I rapidly regained my resting heart rate of 72 and most of my weight of 180.

14. June 7, 2009 Odd pain spot at base of skull on back vanished in a few days. Real but forever a mystery.

15. June 10, 2009 most strenuous hiking (1st PG&E top); no undue stress felt, saw first coyote near parking lot

16. June 14, 2009: at **12 mg**, The confusing Addisonian prednisone-withdrawal symptoms started.

17. June 22, 2009 and 23: a fast trip to the **emergency ward**. In the hospital the prednisone was restored and countless tests revealed nothing apart from age 87. This incident was described in the text.

18. September 17 to October 10 plantar fasciitis left foot; two weeks..

19. October 11, 2009: At **10 mg** I had a flare-up of GCA with fleeting head pains and two inflamed arteries above my right ear, one with a painful spot. **This might have been a catastrophe** if the inflamed artery had been the one supporting my optic nerve.

20. October 30, 2009 Severe hike, 8.5 mile 1000 feet "hit the wall" or "bonk" lost leg strength. This discouraged such hikes.

21. November 2009 to June 2010: unremarkable withdrawal of prednisone from **10mg to 5 mg**.

22. June 1, 2010: taking **5 or 6 mg** and just got back from a long hike in the hills.

23. August 13, 2010: my 89th birthday. I am taking **4 mg** and testing for going down to **3 mg**.

24. September 1, 2010: My doctor declined to order my ESR & CRP lab tests. I requested them and the doctor then ordered them to "make you feel better." The tests were high: ESR=22, CRP=6.6 . On my own, I go back to **4 mg** for another four weeks.

25. October 1, 2010: Constructive appointment with doctor. She ordered continuing ESR-CRP tests and advised staying on a prednisone level for the whole four weeks before the test, saying that one-week on a level before test was not enough.

26. After May 2010: continuing attempts to reduce the prednisone, leading to rising ESR and CRP. High ESR and CRP so prednisone increased to **6 mg** on April 2, 2011. From May 2010 to May 2011 attempts to go below **6 mg**; **5, 4, then 3½ mg** led to rising inflamation as shown by ESR

27. July and August 2011 **legs uncomfortable** -- warning that GCA may be attacking leg arteries. (See Appendix II.)

28. August 29, 2011 – back to **6 mg**.

29. September 14, 2011 – legs feel much better

30. October, November, December 2011 at **7 mg** -- watching my ESR return toward my normal base, less than 10.

31. January 2012 – no symptoms, legs healthy, ESR was 10 on December 29 (Note: the clinic's laboratory erred in reporting 25 on December 26. This shows the importance of the patient keeping good records.)

32. March 2012 – in good health with **5 ½ mg** prednisone daily.

33. April 2012 – in good health with **5 mg** prednisone daily.

34. July 6 to September 12, 2012 – I experienced legs I can best describe as **wearing knee-high boots everywhere too tight**. I continued hiking with no breathlessness or other limit, but avoided the most strenuous climbs

35. August 2012 noticed that tesellopsia was gone. See Appendix IV.

36. January 27, 2016 – I had a 2-day hospitalization with the first appearance of atrial fibrillation. Apart from three years of increasing leg weakness, I'm doing fine. General weakness, for lack of a better description, led to the emergency ward. The diagnosis I can only call "something or other" and the treatment included an oral antibiotic that took several weeks to get out of my bowel.

Six days later my ESR was 40 and my CRP was 20 -- very high for me. Both returned to my normal range after a few days of increased prednisone (**10 mg** quickly tapered to **6 mg**). My guess: these high numbers were not caused by GCA.

I continued the effort to reduce the pjrednisone dosage.

The atrial fibrillation ceased after April 2 but for two eight-hour incidents coincident with GCA symptoms. This raises the question: is there any relation between GCA inflamation and atrial fibrillation? May a slight flare up of GCA trigger fibrillation?

Now down to **4 mg** with no symptoms and hope for further reduction.

Today is August 13, my 95th birthday. Thank you.

One can get to the top of the trail with GCA on 10 mg of prednisone. This 500 feet up a one-mile trail on January 15, 2010 and eleven months of GCA. Over the first five years my hiking and exercise in general decreased. At the age of 95 I must make more effort to get exercise.

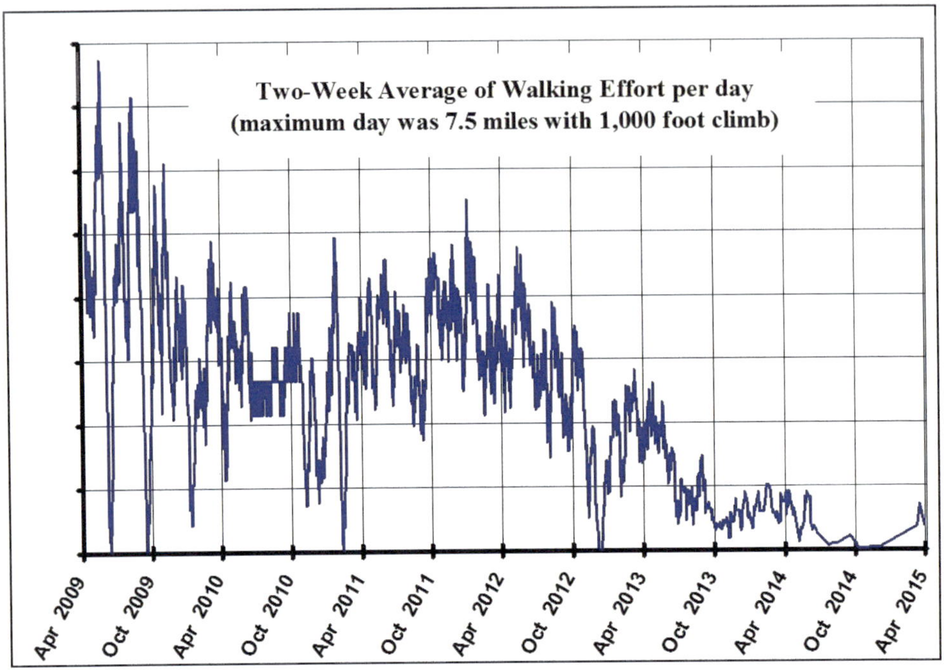

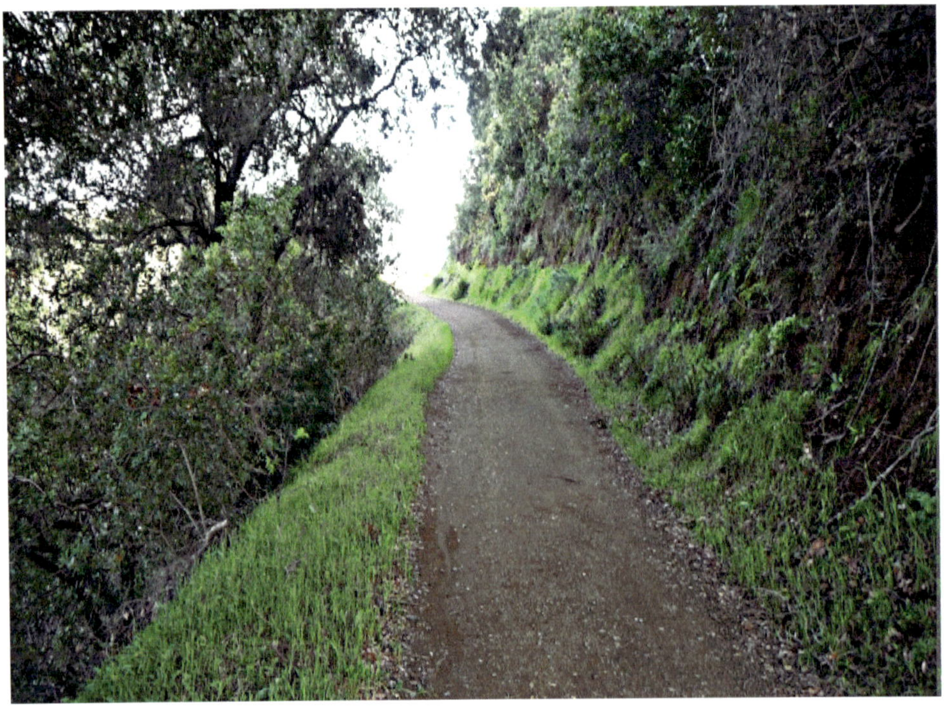

Bibliography

Major clinics offer articles on GCA

Mayo Clinic:

http://www.mayoclinic.com/health/giant-cell-arteritis/ds00440

Cleveland Clinic:

http://my.clevelandclinic.org/disorders/polymyalgia_rheumatica/hic_polymyalgia_rheumatica_and_giant_cell_arteritis_wyntk.aspx

Johns Hopkins:

http://www.hopkinsvasculitis.org/types-vasculitis/giant-cell-arteritis/

The Ophthalmology Department of the University of Iowa hospital and the work of Dr. S Hayreh have been referenced in the text.

http://www.ncbi.nlm.nih.gov/pmc/articles/PMC4314573/

http://webeye.ophth.uiowa.edu/

PubMed offers 6,832 articles from 1940 to August 10, 2016
Most show abstracts, some full articles must be purchased. It may be worthwhile to review the most recent.

http://www.ncbi.nlm.nih.gov/pubmed/?term=temporal+arteritis

The collection by the Norwegians of normal, healthy ESR data was reported here: Journal of Internal Medicine 1996; 240: 125±131

Population-based erythrocyte sedimentation rates in 3910
subjectively healthy Norwegian adults. A statistical study
based on men and women from the Oslo area

http://onlinelibrary.wiley.com/doi/10.1046/j.1365-2796.1996.30295851000.x/full

This Norwegian article refers to Kjeldsberg

" ESR readings "may be especially helpful when the test results are compared with baseline values for the individual patient."

Kjeldsberg CR. Principles of hematological examination. In:
Lee GR, Bithell ThC, Foerster J, Athens JW, Lukens JN, eds.
Wintrobe's Clinical Hematology, Vol. 1, 9th edn. Philadelphia
and London: Lea & Febiger, 1993; 30±2

and to Griffiths, et al:

"... the individually most valid reference is each patient's baseline value judged on the basis of serial recordings."

Griffiths RA, Good WR, Watson NP, O'Donnell HF, Fell PJ,
Shakespeare JM. Normal erythrocyte sedimentation rate in
the elderly. Brit Med J 1984; 289: 724±5.

The response of C-reactive protein and ESR to various infections came from:

British Journal of General Practice, 2004 September 2004 p.653

The course of C-reactive protein response in untreated upper respiratory tract infection
Hasse Melbye, Dag Hvidsten, Arne Holm, Sveine Arne Nordbø, Jan Brox,

Notable is a professional new book made available by Intech:

Advances in the Diagnosis and Treatment of Vasculitis
ISBN: 978-953-307-786-4

http://www.intechopen.com/books/advances-in-the-diagnosis-and-treatment-of-vasculitis

has two chapters that provide much detailed up-to-date information about GCA, intended for reading by specialists. These are best downloaded in .pdf Acrobat format and printed for reading:

http://www.intechopen.com/books/advances-in-the-diagnosis-and-treatment-of-vasculitis/diagnosis-and-treatment-of-giant-cell-arteritis-temporal-arteritis-past-current-and-future-aspects

A short address for this is: http://tinyurl.com/zkd2jt6

Ch. 14 "Diagnosis and Treatment of Giant Cell Arteritis . . ."

Diagnosis and Treatment of Giant Cell Arteritis (Temporal Arteritis) – Past, Current and Future Aspects, Advances in the Diagnosis and Treatment of Vasculitis, Dr. Luis M Amezcua-Guerra (Ed.),

Ch. 15 "Extra-Cranial Manifestations of Giant Cell Arteritis"

Support Groups

There are several support groups on the internet for GCA and PMR. These groups as well as many articles on GCA and PMR may by found by searching the internet.

Participation in such a group may prove valuable, both for medical information and for friendly support.

A friendly and helpful group is the United Kingdom PMR and GCA Forum.

http://pmrandgca.myfunforum.org

with more than 50 very smart and PMR-experienced members:

The United Kingdom has many local support groups this forum can help you contact..

A valuable US support group is:

https://groups.yahoo.com/neo/groups/pmrusa/info

A member of that group, JamesWRupp has collected countless references and much information about GCA. Join one or more of these groups and exchange experiences.

Appendix I – Leg Discomfort Incident

My leg discomfort was real but hard to describe. The best I could tell my doctor was that my legs "felt stiff." I've learned to describe the feeling as "wearing knee-high boots that are too tight everywhere." I have used the expressions, "walking on the legs of Frankenstein's monster" or "walking on stilts." "Painful" did not apply. There was no pain.

Leg pain may be caused by claudication – poor blood circulation. But standard-grade claudication causes increased discomfort with exercise. My legs would walk as far as I wished with no increase in discomfort. They did discourage me from taking my longer walks – perhaps for fear of walking into a problem.

Perhaps it was the lack of typical claudication symptoms that caused me to largely dismiss the leg discomfort as being related to GCA or a prednisone side-effect. This went on for more than two months – until the morning I saw my black-and-blue heel.

Putting on my socks I noticed that my left heel was black and blue. I do not recall if this was true for my right heel. My first thought was dye stain from my black socks. Dumb idea – my socks were old, washed with whites many time and had no dye to stain my heel. Nevertheless, I scrubbed the heel to remove the black-and-blue color, to no avail. I made a second dumb error by not photographing the heel – I photograph everything else. Then I made a third dumb error. I should have taken my heel directly to the clinic for examination – for the record if nothing else.

What is did do was swallow an extra 5 mg prednisone pill and increase my daily schedule from 5 mg to 6 mg. My legs and my heel became normal in a few days or two weeks. To be safe, after one month I increased to 7 mg for the next three months. I sought safe ground.

I regret not having my legs and black-and-blue heel examined by a doctor.

Appendix II – Tesellopsia Hallucination

During my hiking expeditions, I often, if not always, saw what I later learned to be a hallucination called "tesellopsia" – below is a poor depiction of the black screen that blocked my path. It first appeared on the uphill side only, later on both sides and in front of me. I simply walked through it. Trying to examine it caused it to disappear. The doctor called it "migraneous" but I called if amusing. It appeared only during serious climbing and disappeared on the downhill return. Induced apparently by exercise, although I was never breathless in the slightest. It disappeared sometime in 2012 relataive to nothing. The usual suspects: GCA, prednisone, or prednisone withdrawal.

Note: I have had no eye problems, My vision has always been good.

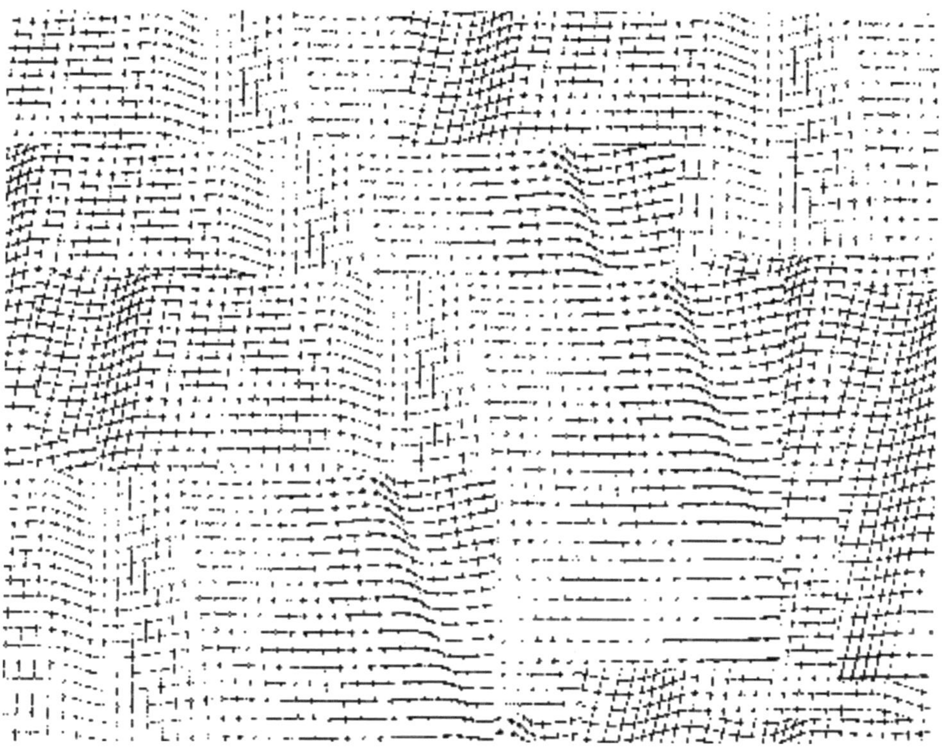

Appendix III – The Cost of GCA

I find reading Medicare reports difficult. This is my best effort of summarizing my GCA medical costs, listed as the Medicare-approved amounts (much less than the "charged" amounts). I claim no accuracy. However, I believe the basics are correct. Diagnosis is costly mainly because of confusing symptoms that require examination of various possibilities. In my case:

1. The dry cough that may have had nothing to do with this story
2. The two symptoms unrelated to GCA that suggested need for a brain scan and a colonoscopy – the latter probably a good idea anyway.

Costs of the treatment of GCA consists of doctor visits and prednisone, neither of which is terribly expensive.

However, an event compelling emergency care – hospitalization – can be costly. Even if for only two days if a cardiac intensive-care facility is deemed necessary.

GCA Diagnosis	Dry cough	$ 2,100
	Primary care doctor and tests	$ 2,100
	Brain scan	$ 520
	Colonoscopy	$ 3,000
GCA Treatment	Rheumatologist and tests	$ 1,600
	First Hospitalization	$ 32,000
	Ophthalmology	$ 320
	Prednisone	$ 300
	DEXA bone scan (2)	$ 150

I was retired and and paying for supplementary insurance and under-paying for Medicare. In addition to the cost of two insurances my cash out-of-pocket cost was about $1,400 and about $300 for prednisone. Without insurance the cost would have been prohibitive. I could not have afforded to have GCA – certainly not if I were to crash into the hospital.

For its own reasons Medicare later decided it would not pay the $32,000 for the first hospitalization, Consequently the hospital had to return my copay of $1,800. Both I and the hospital appealed without success. Apparently Medicare thought the hospital did too much. Makes limited sense.

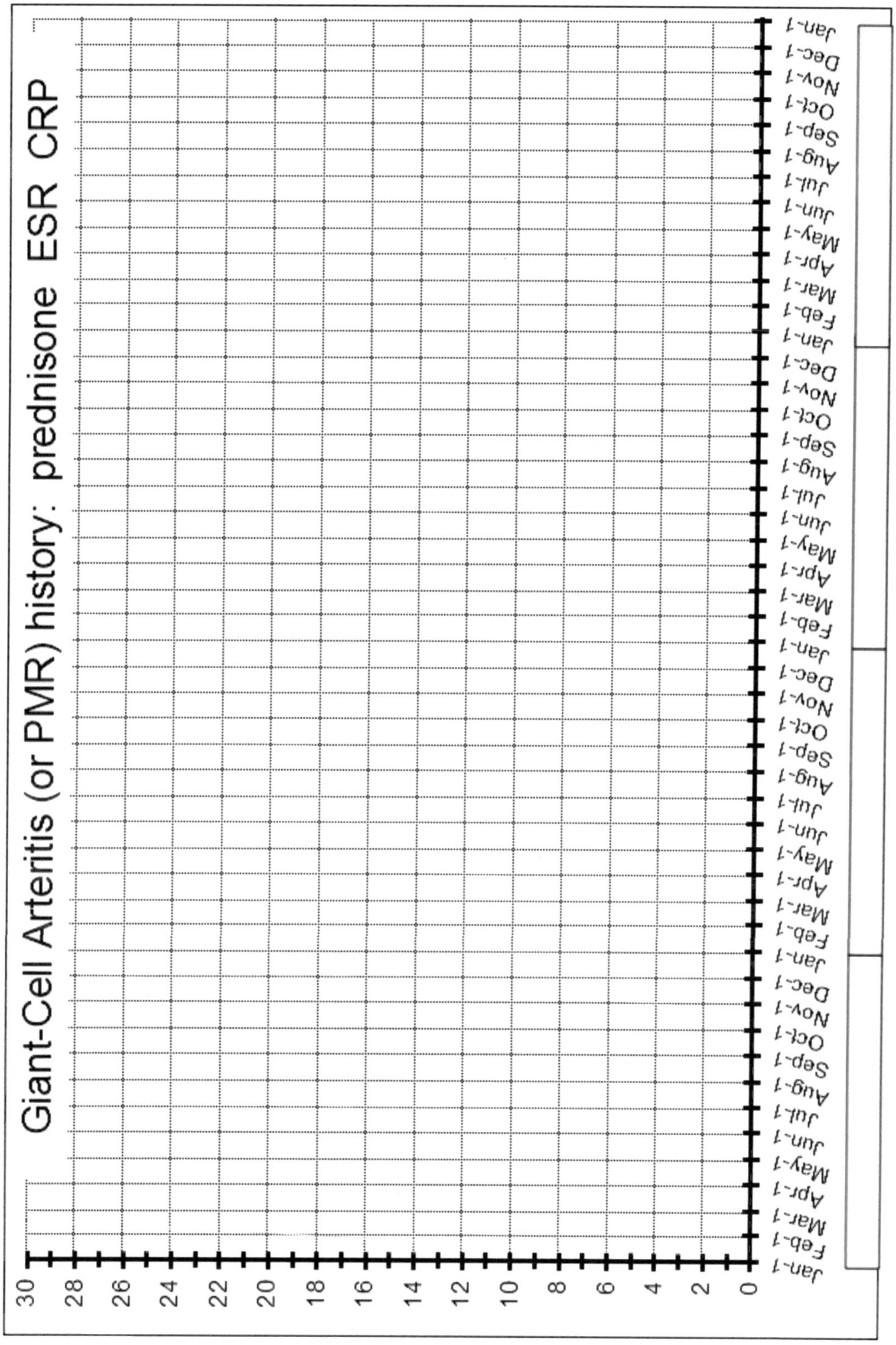
Giant-Cell Arteritis (or PMR) history: prednisone ESR CRP
30 28 26 24 22 20 18 16 14 12 10 8 6 4 2 0
Jan-1 Feb-1 Mar-1 Apr-1 May-1 Jun-1 Jul-1 Aug-1 Sep-1 Oct-1 Nov-1 Dec-1 Jan-1 Feb-1 Mar-1 Apr-1 May-1 Jun-1 Jul-1 Aug-1 Sep-1 Oct-1 Nov-1 Dec-1 Jan-1 Feb-1 Mar-1 Apr-1 May-1 Jun-1 Jul-1 Aug-1 Sep-1 Oct-1 Nov-1 Dec-1 Jan-1 Feb-1 Mar-1 Apr-1 May-1 Jun-1 Jul-1 Aug-1 Sep-1 Oct-1 Nov-1 Dec-1 Jan-1

Made in United States
Troutdale, OR
11/03/2026

56844707R00029